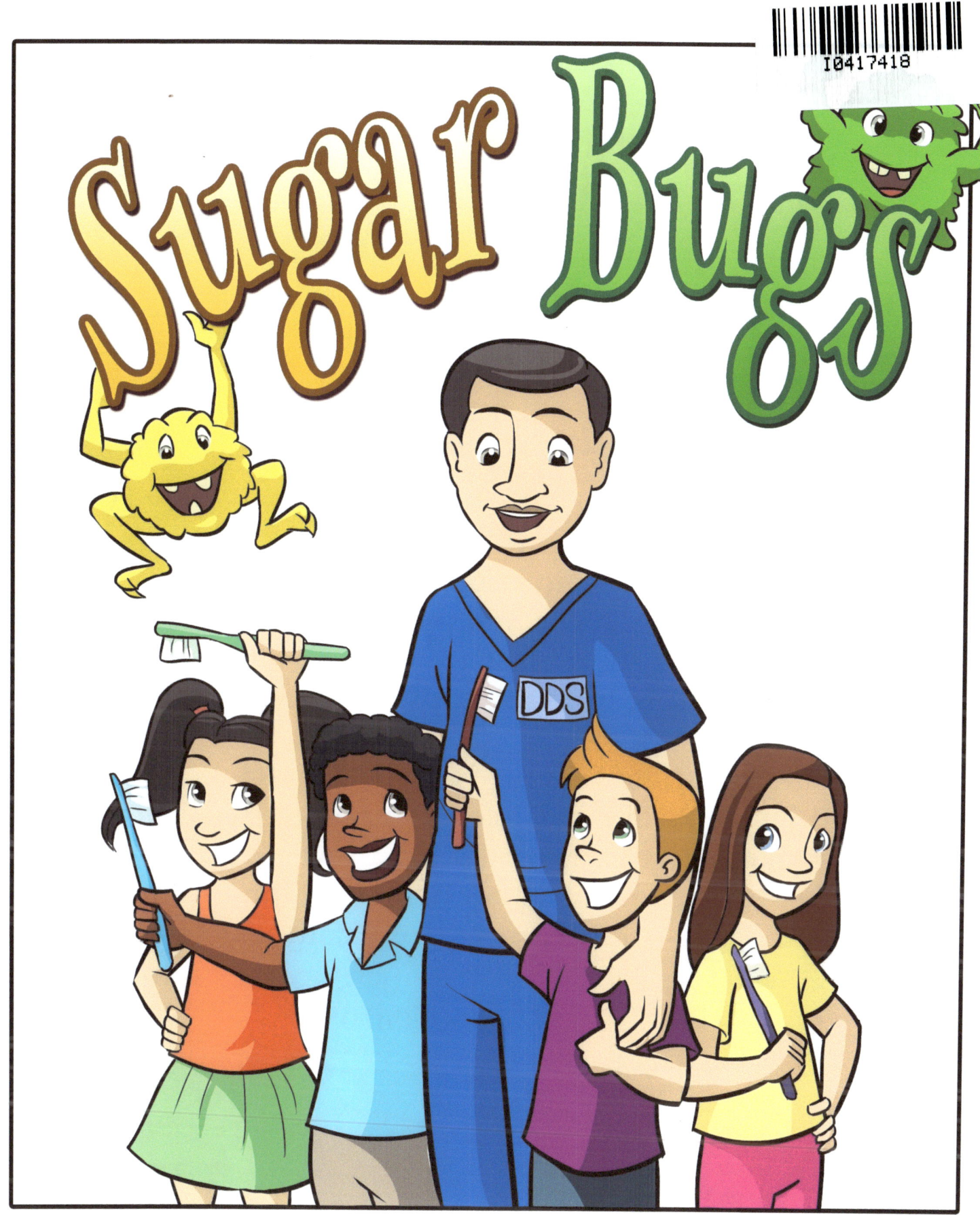

Sugar Bugs

Written by
Roberto N. Loar DDS

Illustrated by
Marvin Alonso

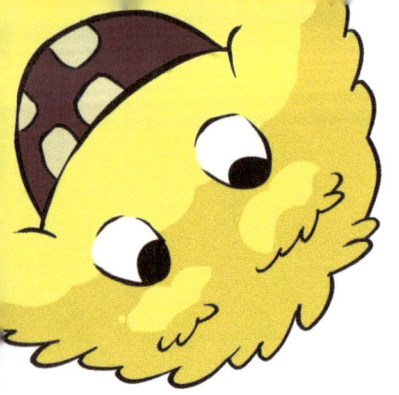

Sugar Bugs

Copyright © 2017 by Roberto N. Loar DDS

ISBN 978-1539067054

This book is dedicated to

Children of all ages who wish to have a happy and healthy smile!

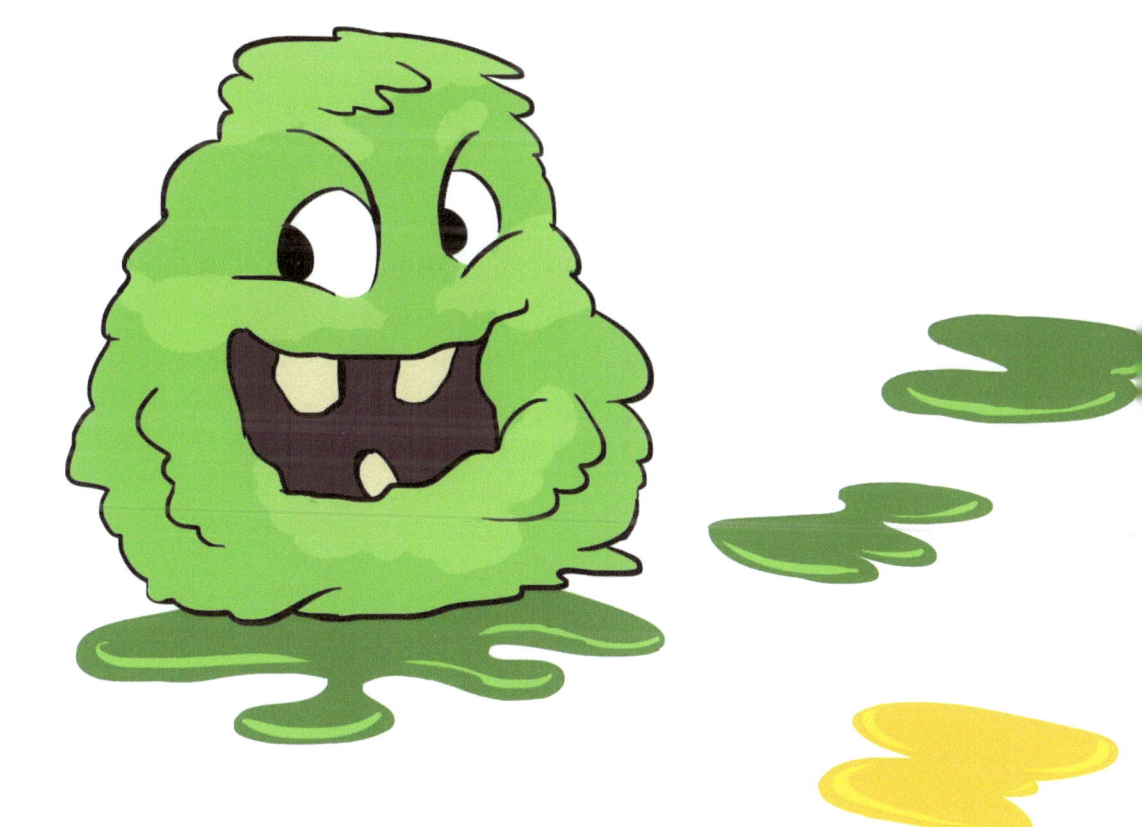

Sugar bugs are tiny, small,

and they happen to live in the mouths of us all.

Even though they are too small to see,

they stay in the mouths of Mommy, Daddy, you, and me.

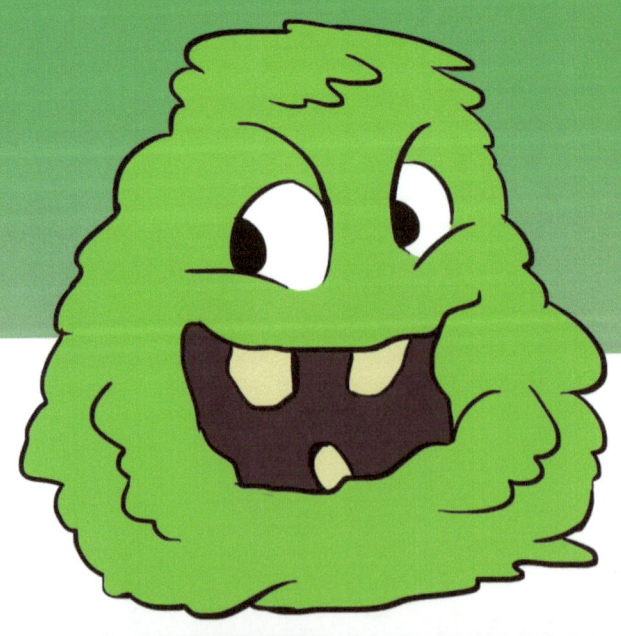

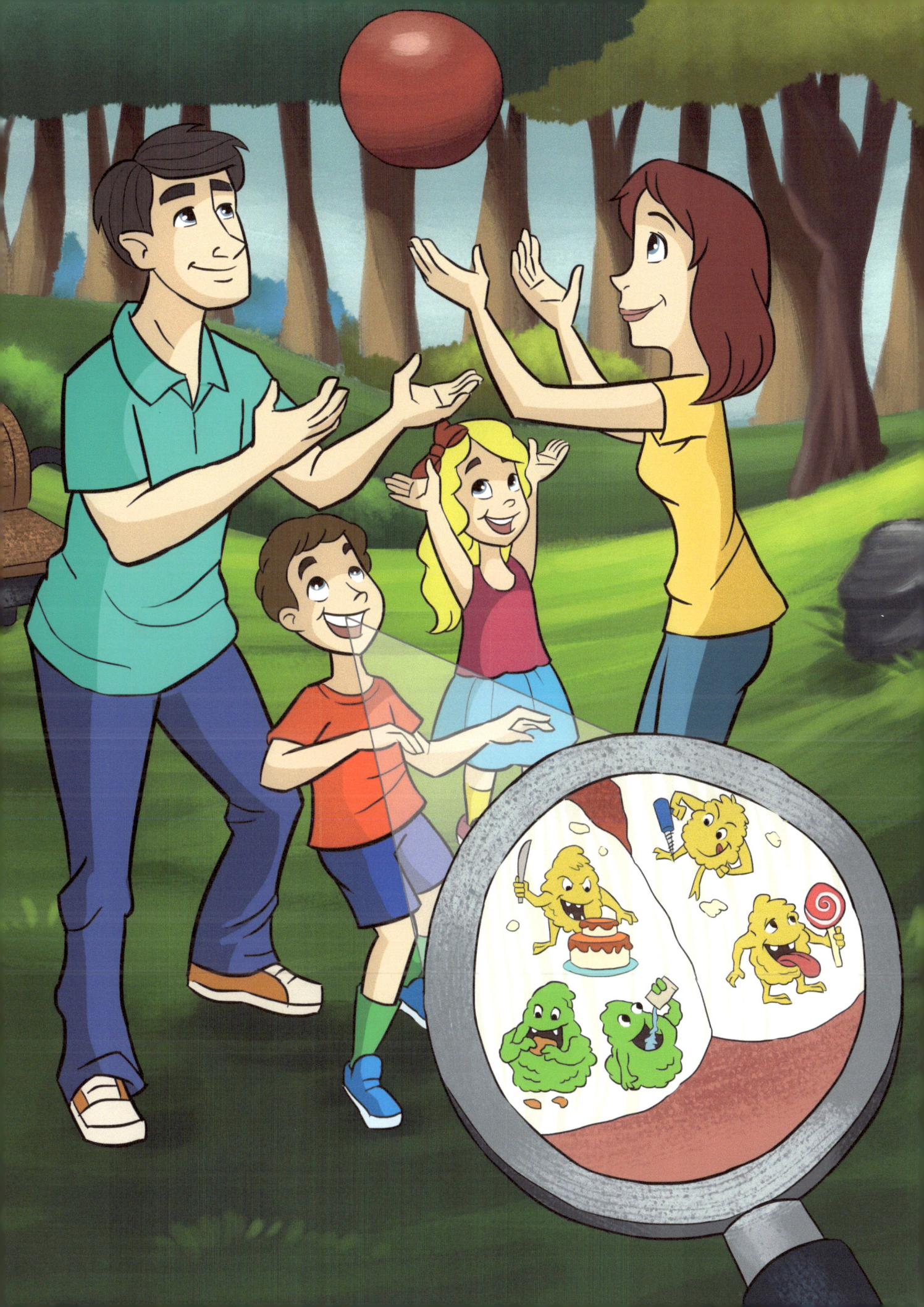

Now, can you guess what these sugar bugs eat?

Sugar, of course; they eat everything sweet.

Sugar is in candies, cookies, and desserts galore;

so when you drink sodas, the sugar bugs eat more.

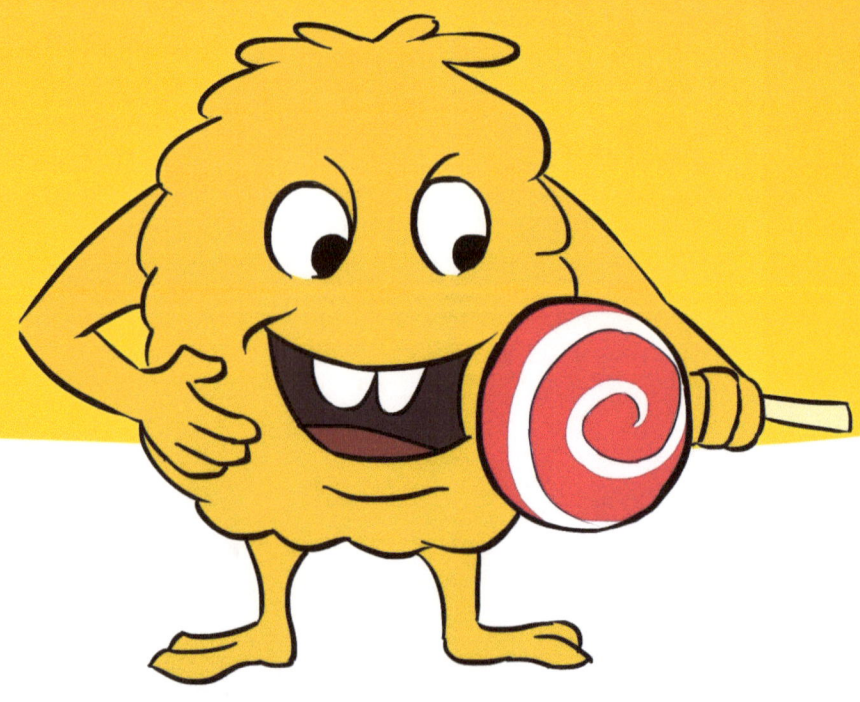

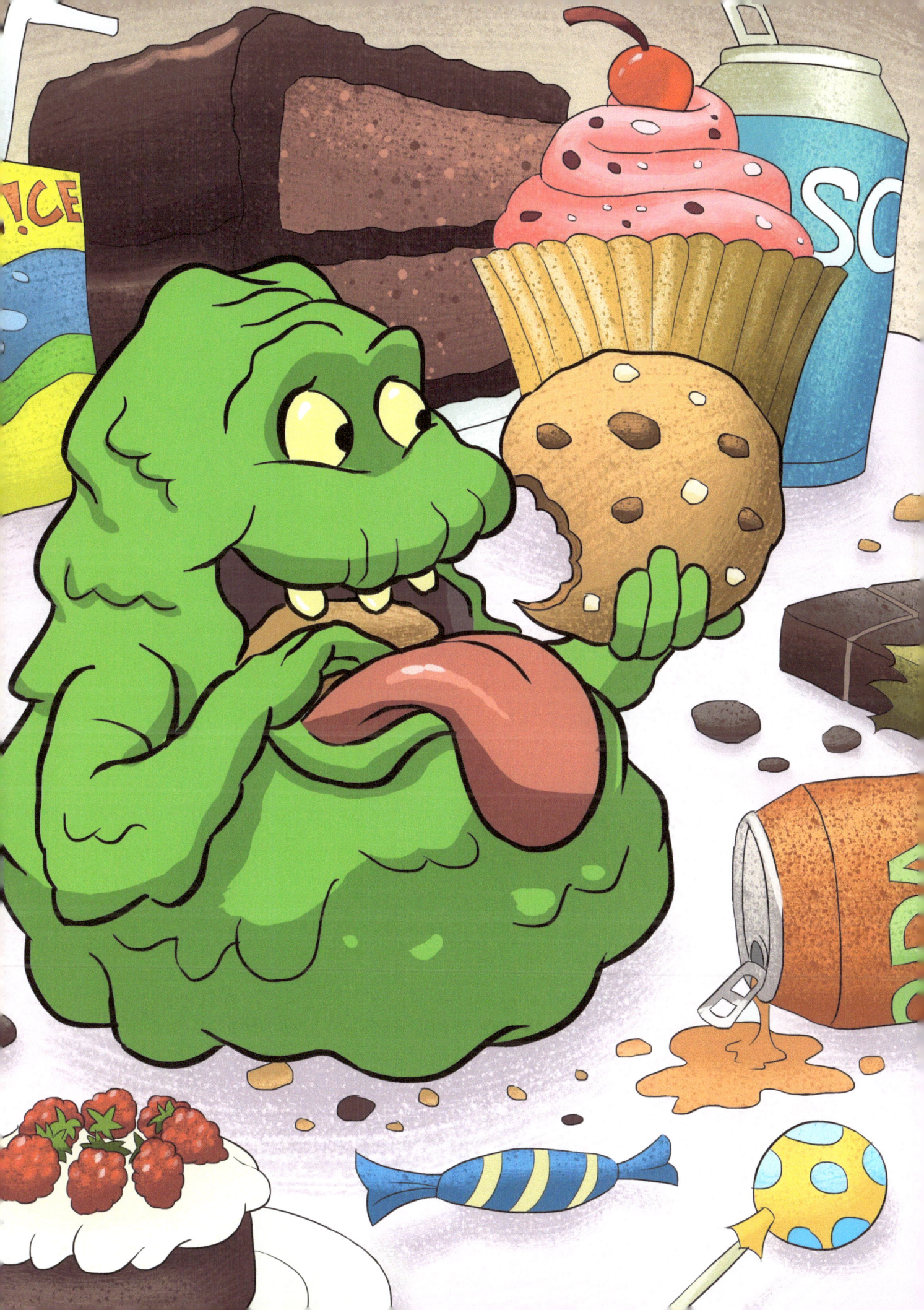

The problem comes with what the sugar bugs do.

When they are full of sugar, then they pee and they poo.

They live in this mess that sticks to your teeth,

and if they keep growing, they give you much grief.

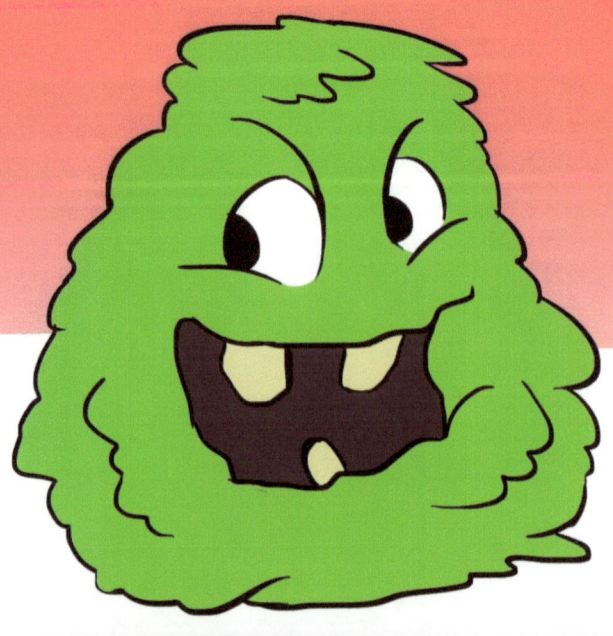

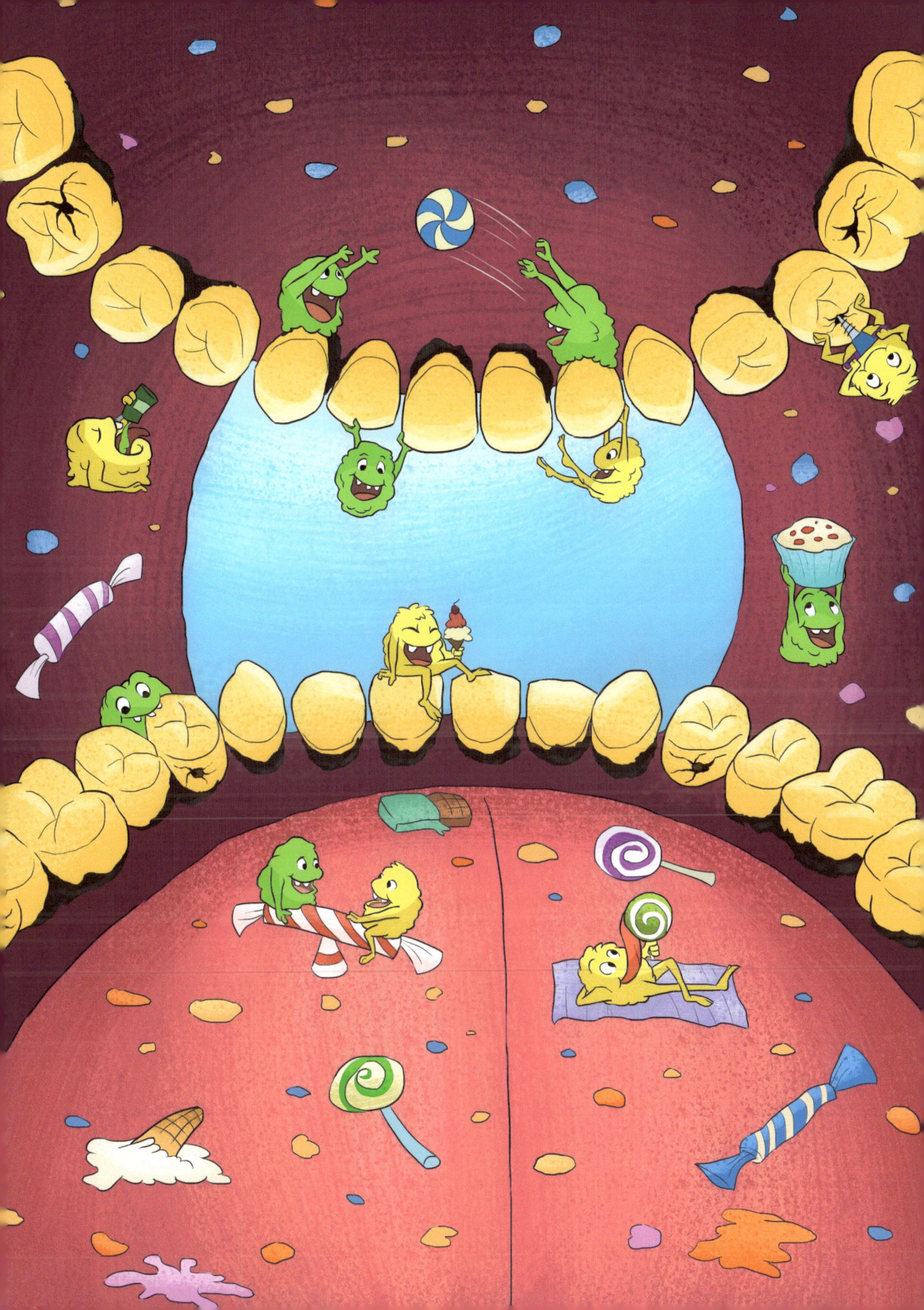

After a while they make
your teeth as weak as can be,
and you get a little black hole
called a cavity.
Now, once you get that, it's a
little too late;
but you can go to the dentist,
and he'll fix you up straight.
He can clean out the bugs and
all the decay
and then put in a filling that
very same day.

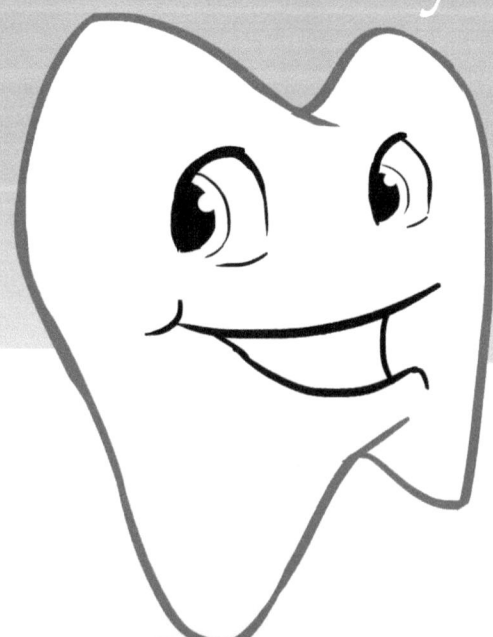

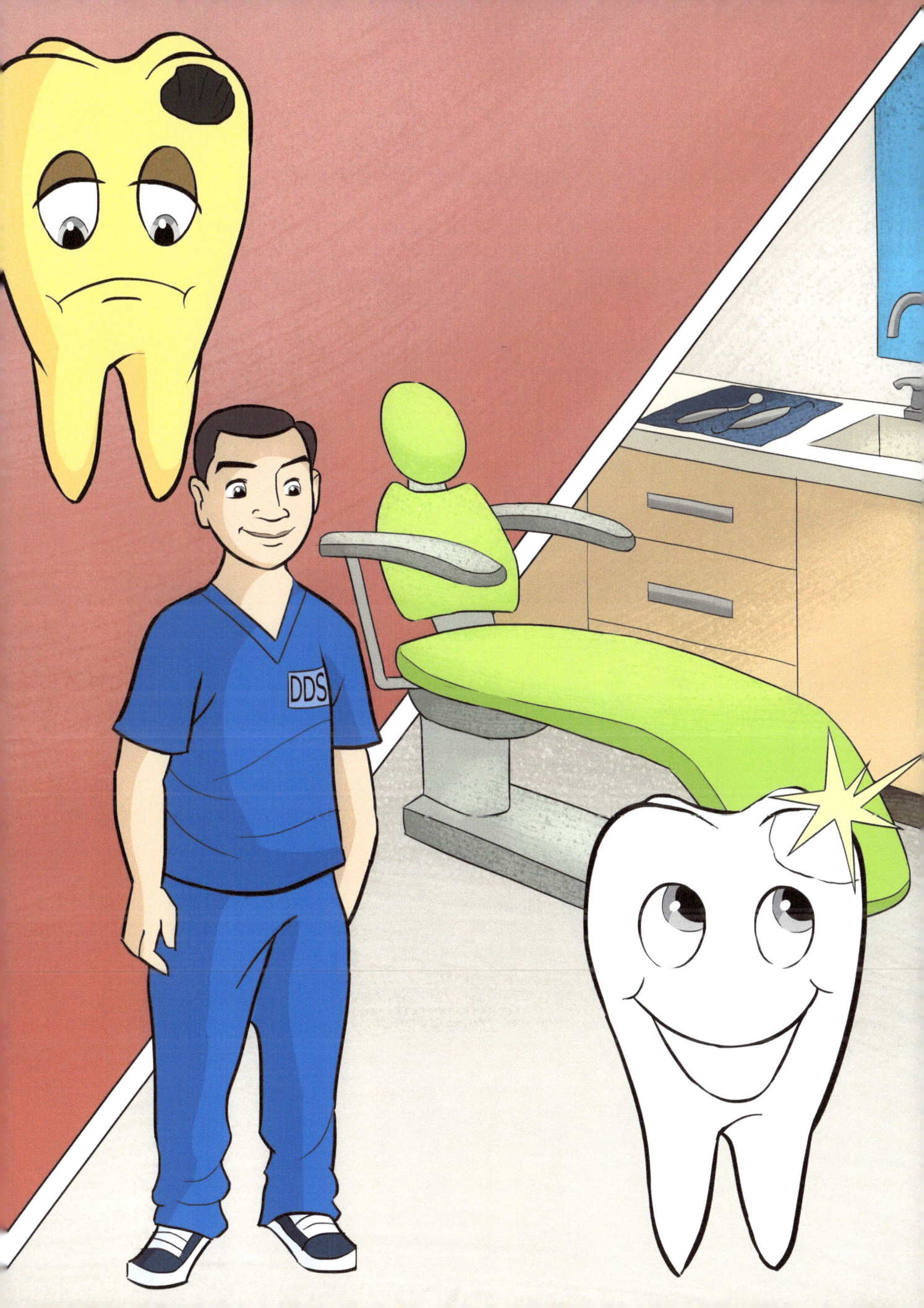

Now here is the question,
what can you do?
You don't want any sugar bugs
with their pee and their poo.
The first step is to start with
what the bugs eat.
We need to cut back on cookies,
candies, and sweets.
Put down that soda and drink
water instead.
Then the sugar bugs can't eat
and they become dead.

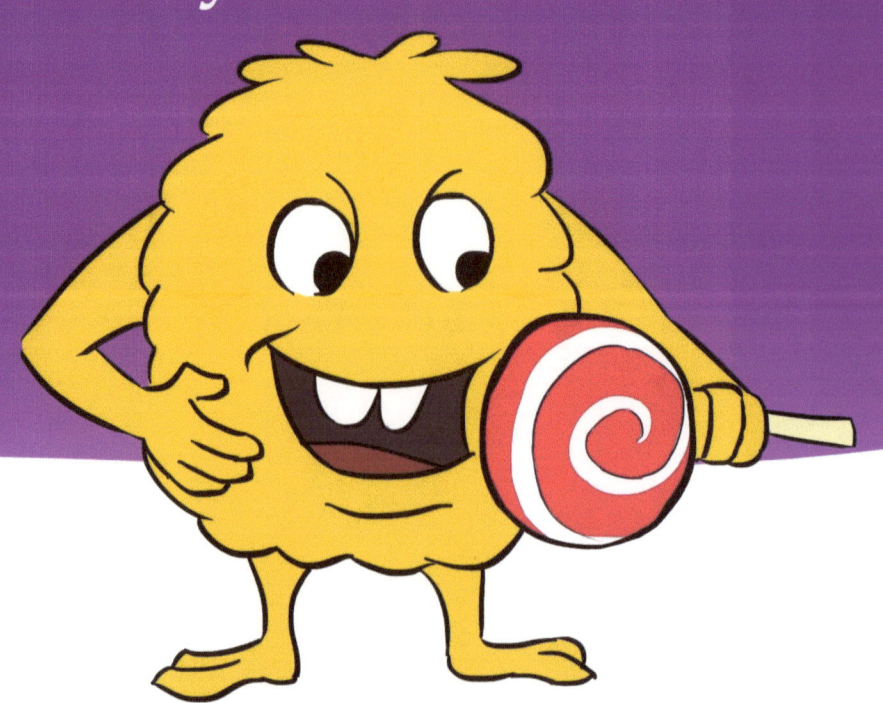

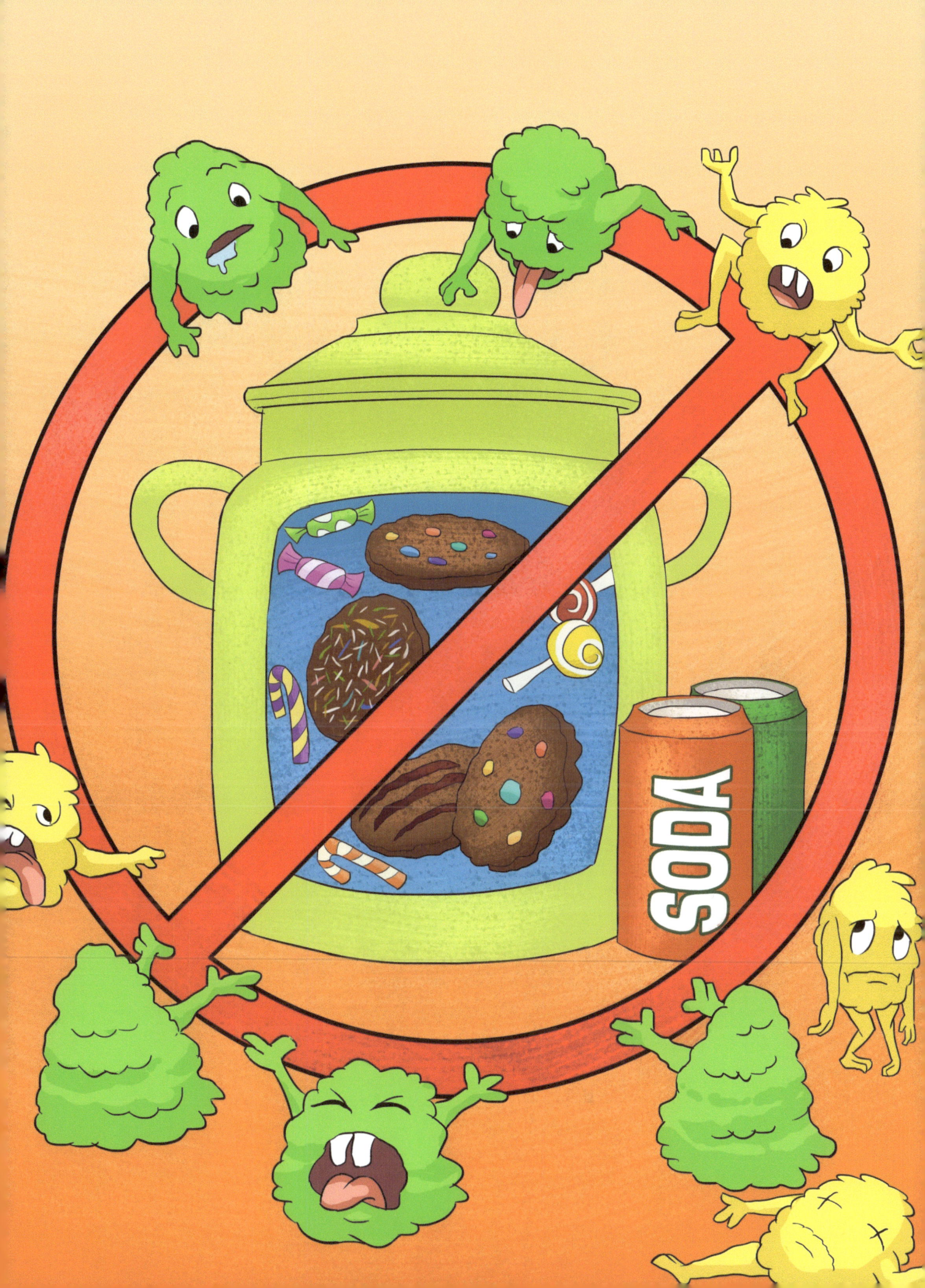

The second step is as important as one.
It's about cleaning your teeth, and it can be fun.
Let's start with when: morning and night.
Two times a day will keep your smile bright.

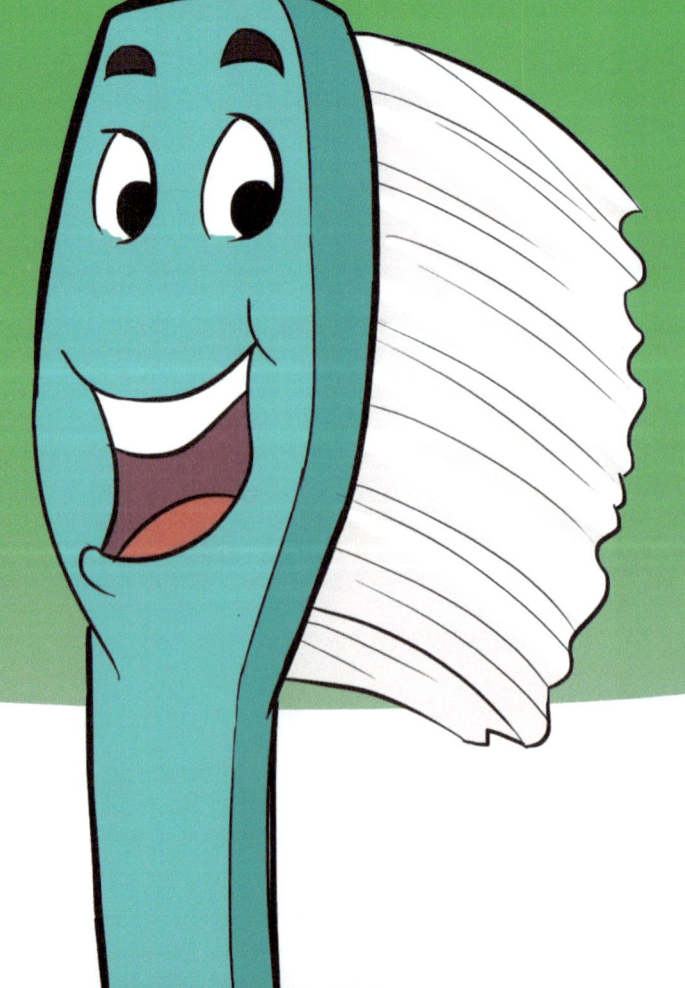

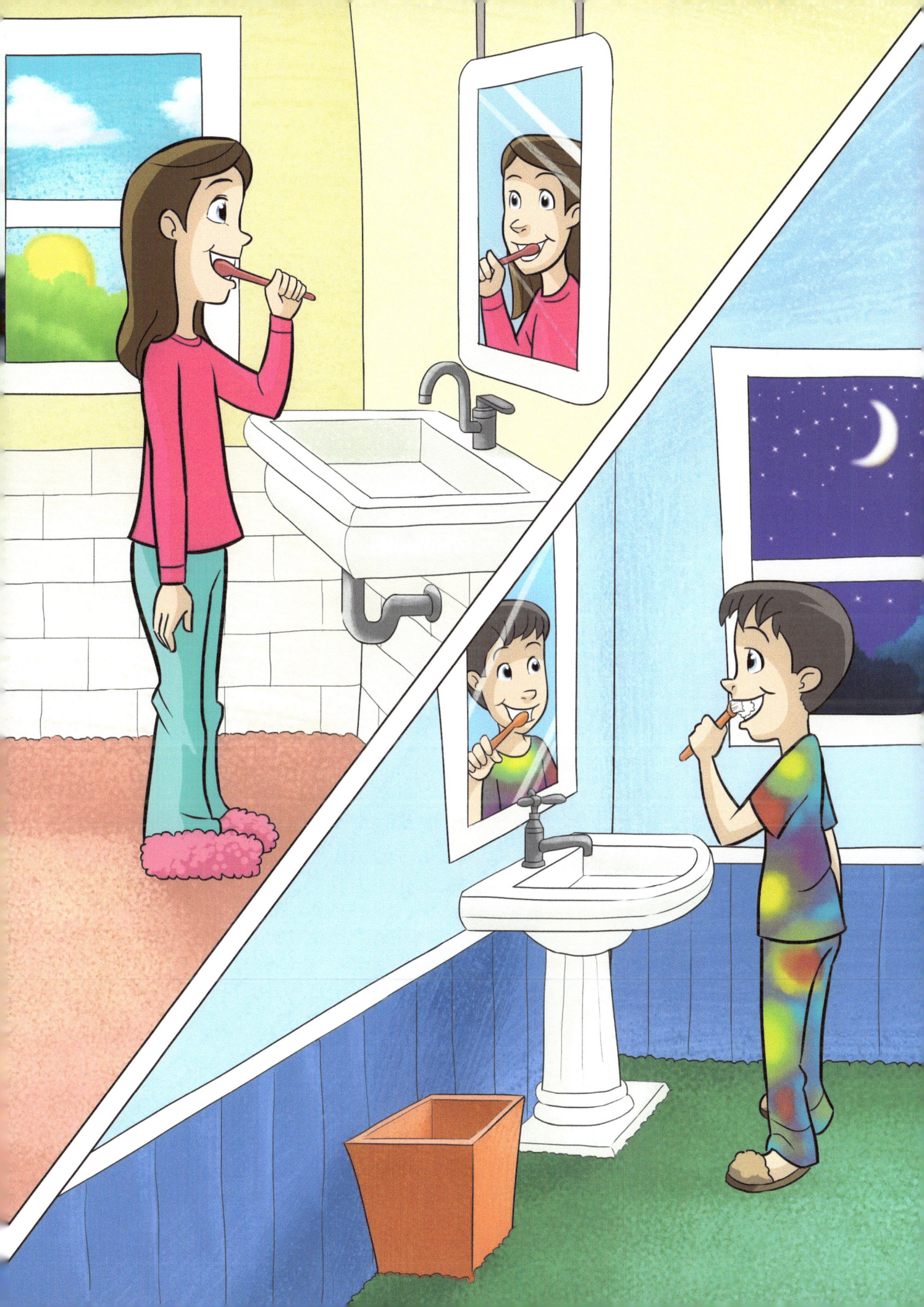

Put toothpaste on your brush, not more than a drop.

Remember to get the teeth on their front, back, and top.

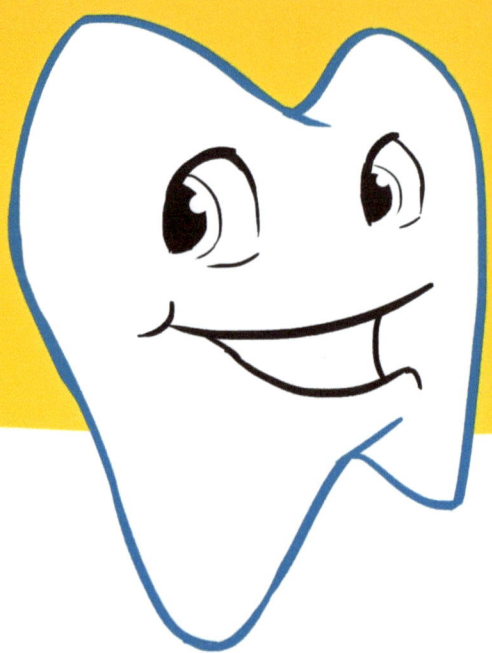

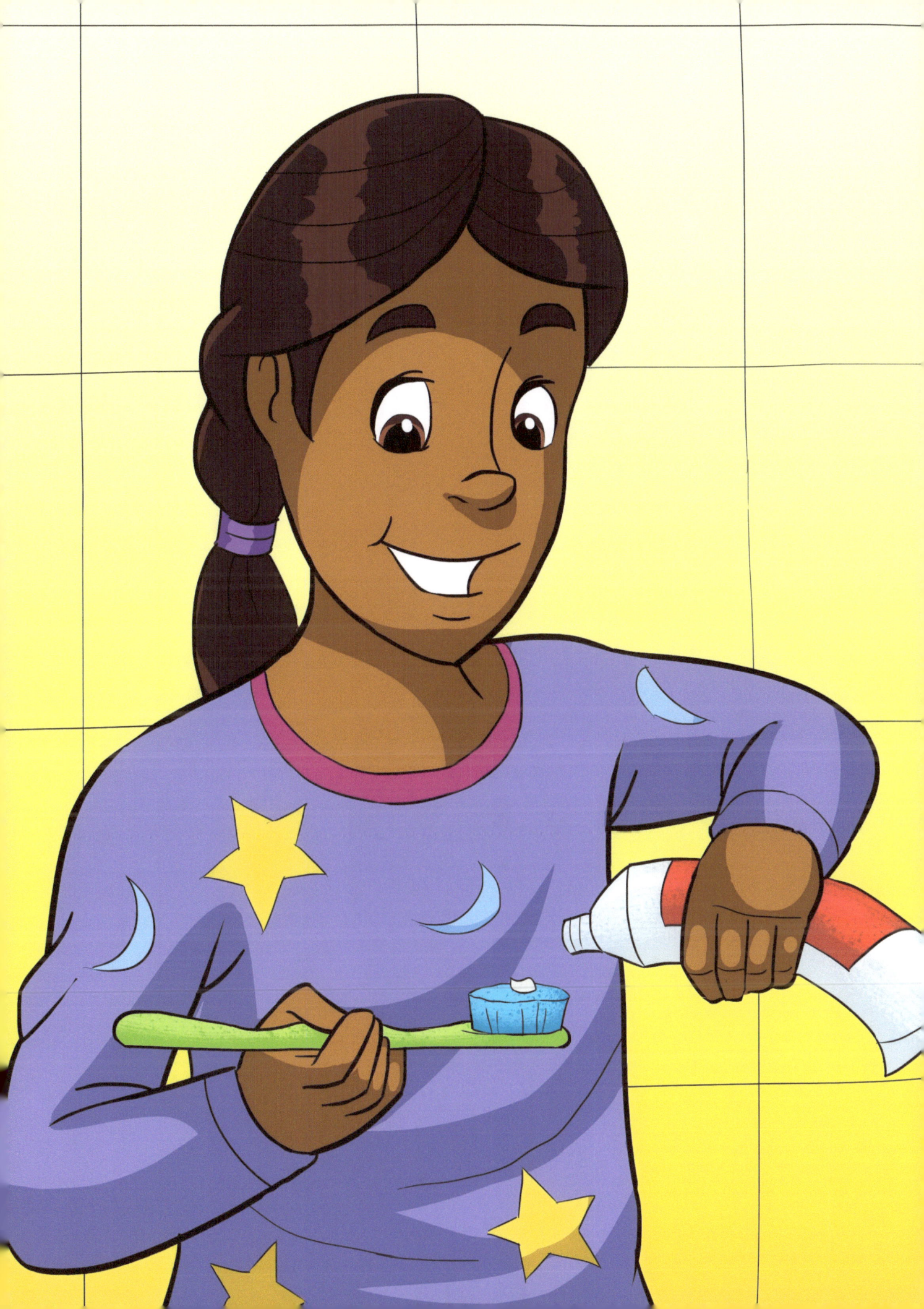

Make little circles; start in the back and go 'round. Be sure not to stop until every tooth has been found.

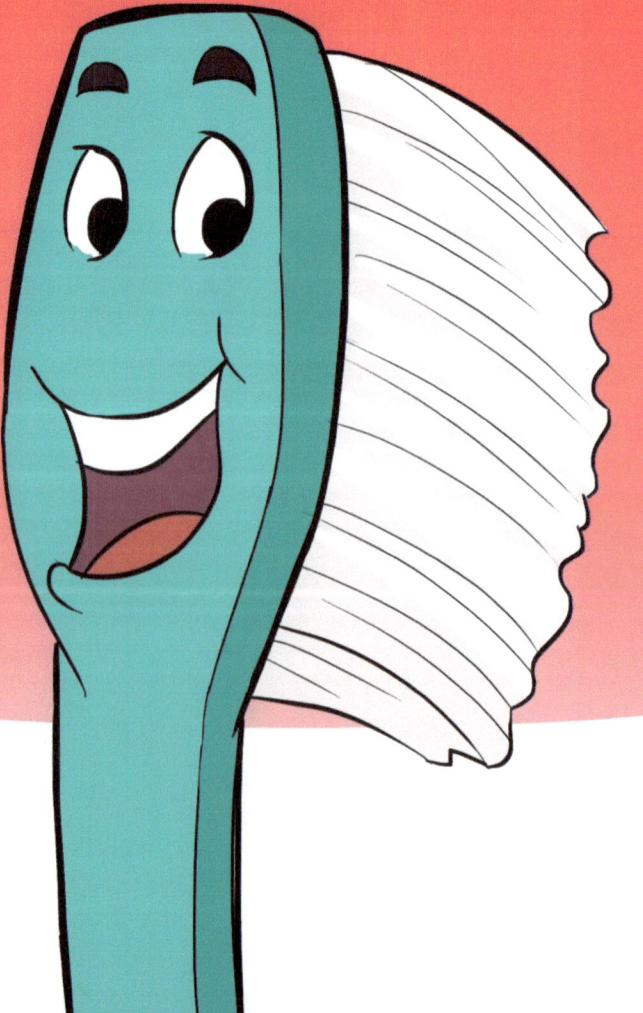

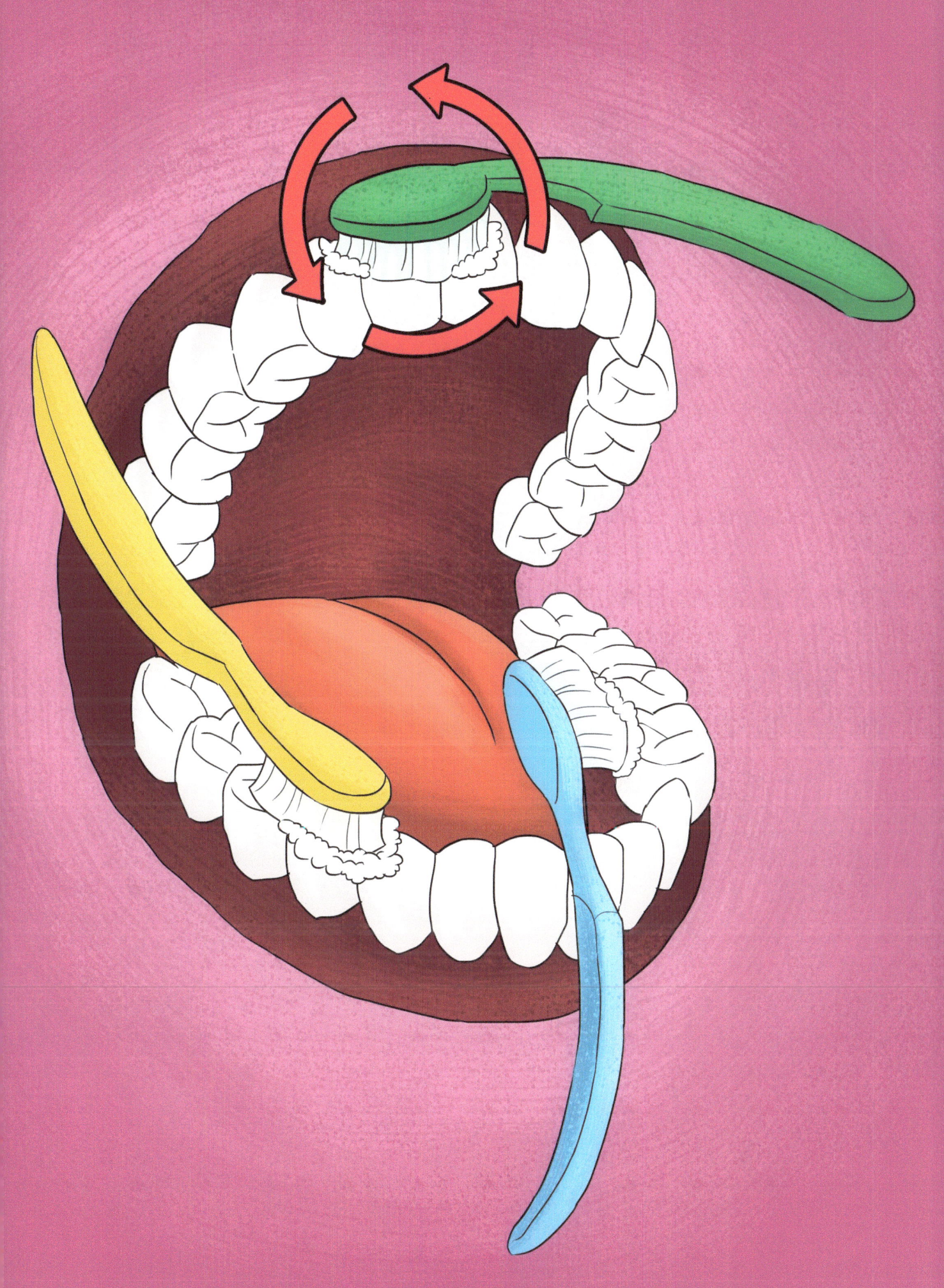

And just so your teeth
never get sad,
floss and mouthwash are
two things you can add.

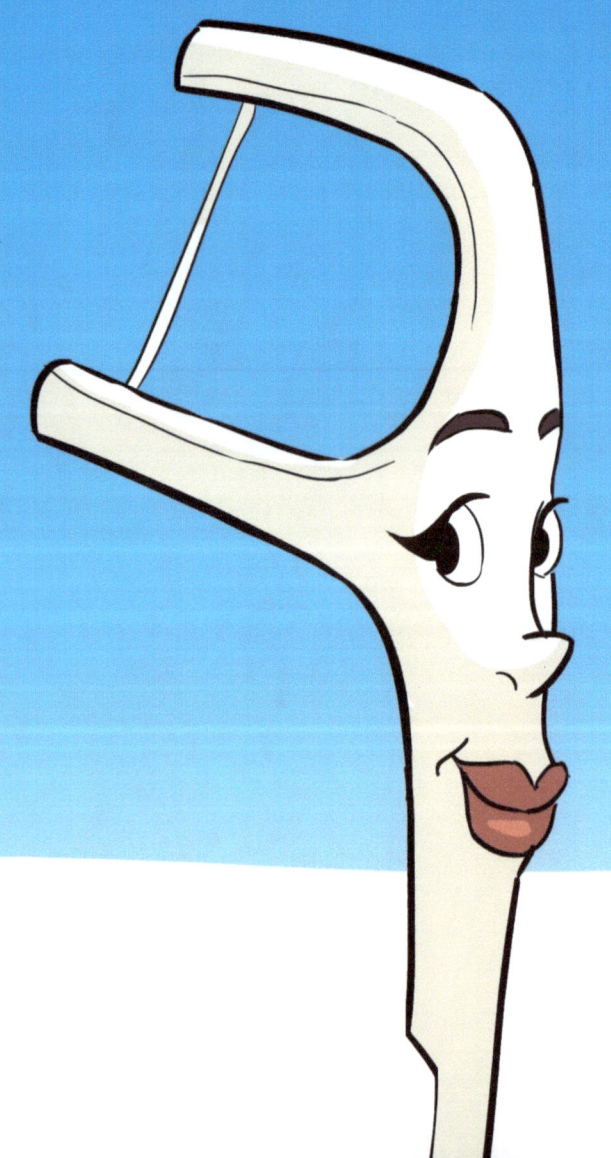

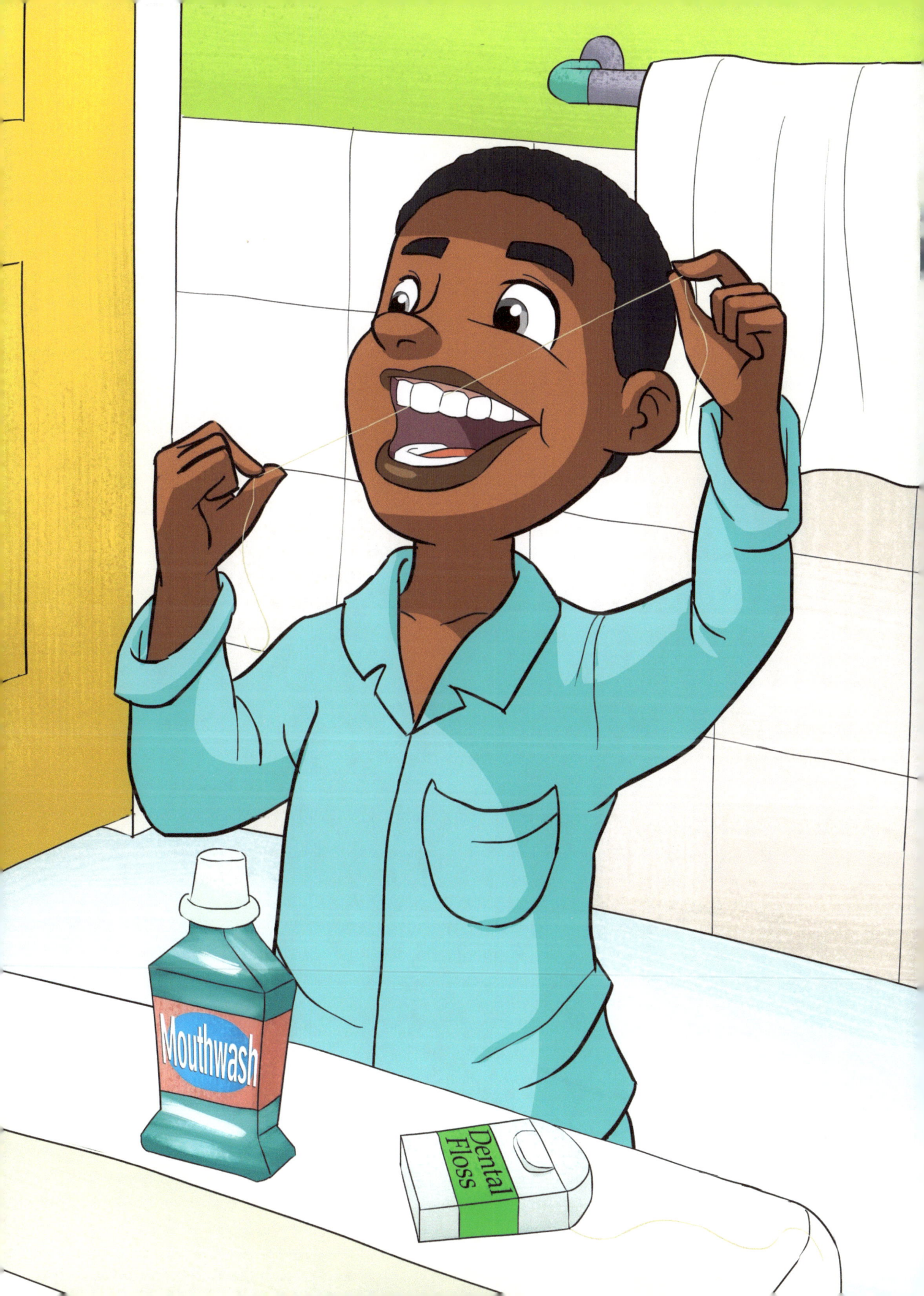

The last step is one that I truly hold dear.
Be sure to see your dentist at least two times a year.

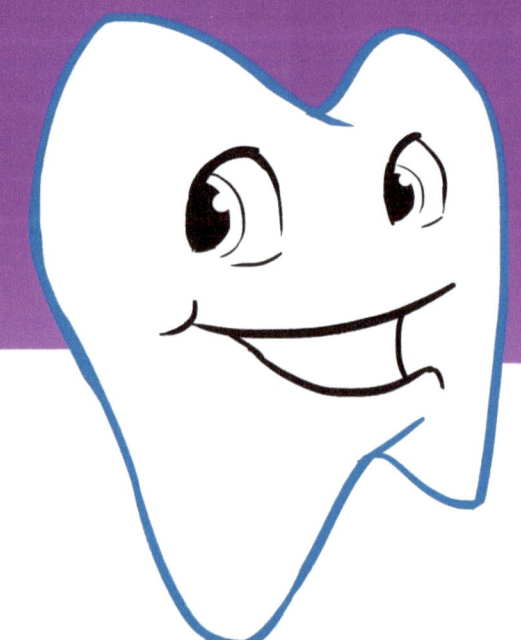

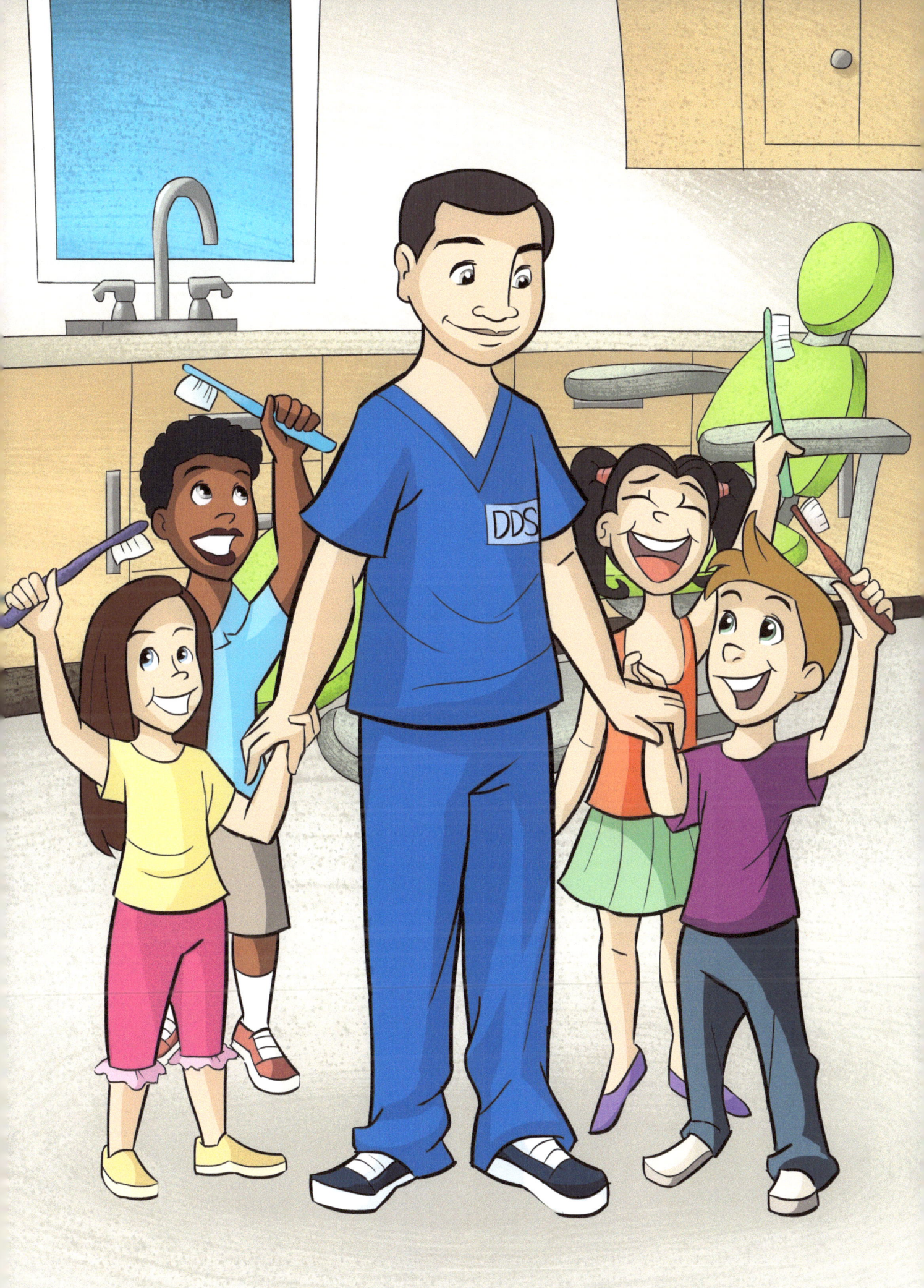

The End

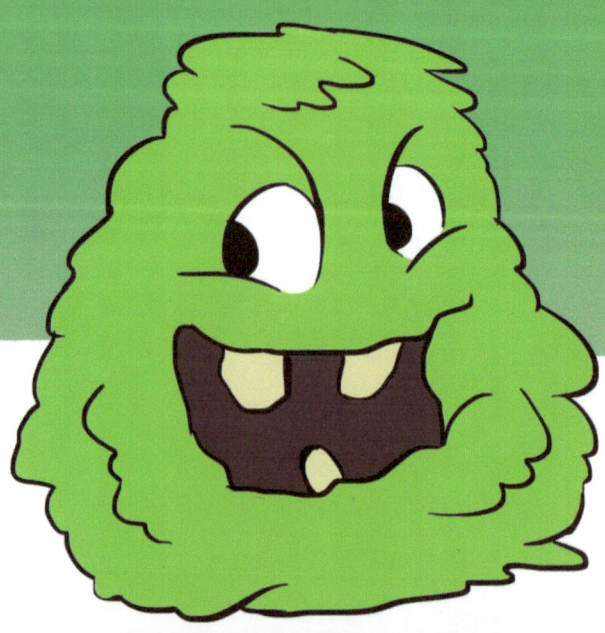

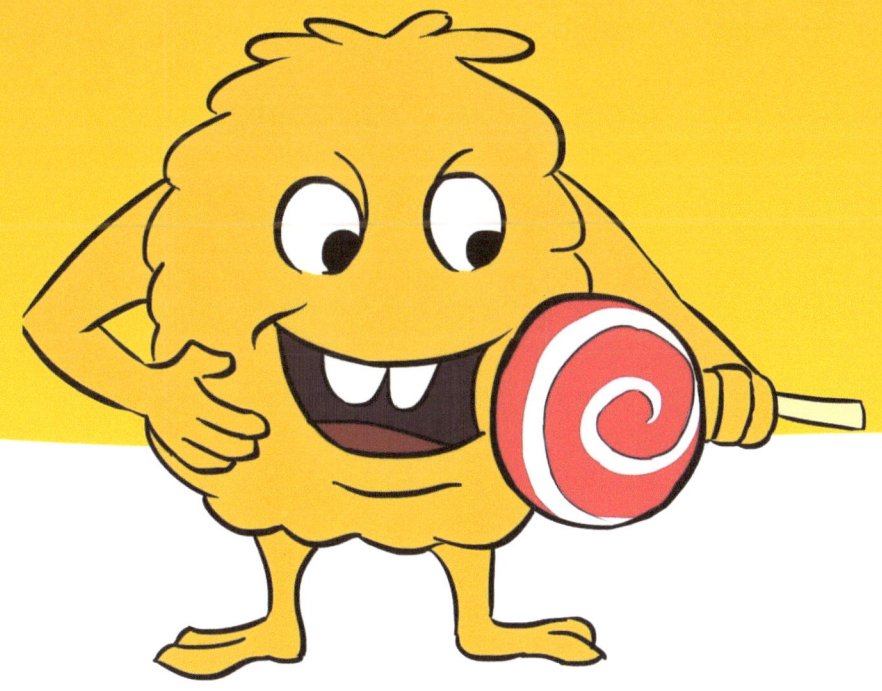

www.ingramcontent.com/pod-product-compliance
Lightning Source LLC
Chambersburg PA
CBHW060827290526
45792CB00005BB/1828